RETHINKING DIABETES

A VERY PERSONAL INVESTIGATION
INTO THE UNDERLYING CAUSES OF
DIABETES, WITH A NEW VIEW TOWARDS
TREATMENT AND CARE, PLUS PROSPECTS
FOR AN EVENTUAL GLOBAL ERADICATION.

By Bud Kuhlmann

ISBN 978-1-312-35568-2

9 781312 355682

90000

RETHINKING DIABETES

I ask the reader to please keep in mind that this book is only concerning Type Two diabetes. After writing this book a friend encouraged me to investigate Type One diabetes. Type One diabetes is related but has very different causes and should be treated by medical professionals in a very different manner than the things mentioned in this book.

In addition, while reading about Type One Diabetes, it is the author's opinion that Type One diabetes is probably preventable, but that such a bold discovery in that regard is left for others and is out of the realm of my study and understanding.

DISCLAIMER: The author of this book is not a medical professional. This book is for informational purposes only. The reader is strongly urged to seek medical consultation and supervision before even considering actions based upon this book. The information in this book has not been reviewed by any medical professional, and it might be entirely wrong information. Enjoy the book and consider its message but do not act upon this information in any manner. With the AMA in mind, the author assumes no liability if anybody foolishly ignores this disclaimer.

CHAPTER ONE

SELF-EXPERIMENTATION LEADS TO UNCOMMON CONCLUSIONS ABOUT TYPE TWO DIABETES

July 14, 2014

It is time for the medical world to revisit that most dreaded plague: Diabetes.

I, the author of this book have been a type two diabetic for almost my entire life, having failed a blood sugar test at age 16. Before explaining the truth about diabetes, I wish to give a brief history of my research into this matter.

Having watched my mother succumb to diabetes, I noted that her dietary efforts and her strict insulin regimen both failed to cure the diabetes and failed to stop the progressive deterioration. Having a leg amputated due to circulatory failure at age sixty, her health declined rapidly and she died at age sixty-three, obeying her doctor's instructions all the way to the grave.

Determined to not go the same route as my mother, I chose to go through life experimenting with my health sans medical treatments of any kind. I ate regular foods, took no medications, and for the most part, allowed the diabetes to ravage my body. For over thirty years, I attempted to control the diabetes and its symptoms by original methods based solely upon my personal decades-long observations and experiments.

Most people do not take it upon themselves to experiment with their health as I have, but for me, it is always exciting and educational. Confident in my ability to experiment on my body, I began doing all of the things which diabetics are warned against. I would live on ice cream for a weekend, drink sugary sodas for months at a time, eat pies and cakes and just do everything commonly shunned by diabetics. And the interesting thing was that I eventually started noticing patterns. I started to become wise to the ways diabetes affected the body.

I, of course, wrecked my health. My blood sugar was often over 400 for weeks on end, and yet I knew that taking medicines and listening to diabetic doctors would at best alleviate the symptoms and perhaps extend my life as a miserable diabetic. I knew that diabetic medicine dealt mostly with alleviating the symptoms. I was after a cure; a fix. For forty years, I lived as an untreated diabetic, trusting in my instincts and trying all sorts of disapproved behaviors and self-treatments.

But all of this was about to change for the better, and largely because I moved to Florida.

In Florida, a neighbor of mine had a large orange tree. His tree produced many hundreds of oranges each year, and most of them just fell to the ground and attracted rats. He agreed that I could have them all, and so the idea of living for a week exclusively upon orange juice became an instant plan for experimental action.

Each day, I would hand-squeeze two to three gallons of wonderful, fresh orange juice, and I drink it all the same day that it was squeezed. I was using my blood sugar meter and test strips daily to monitor my blood sugar levels. After only about three days, it became clear to me that my blood sugar level was dropping by over twenty points per day. At the end of the week, my blood sugar levels had gone from about four hundred to a level below two hundred and fifty. I was astonished; I was astonished and I felt wonderful.

Every year for the next 12 years, I would harvest the fully ripe oranges in mid-January and begin my orange juice 'fasting' diet. I would diet intentionally for 21 days every year. Here is what would happen every time:

After about fifteen days on the orange juice plan, my blood sugar would plateau at about 90. It never went below that level. By concentrated monitoring of my blood sugar, I could see that my blood sugar was around 90 before drinking a large glass of orange juice. As an experiment, I'd drink 32 ounces of orange juice in ten minutes, wait fifteen minutes, and test my blood sugar levels again. It was usually a jump of twenty to fifty points. A final test thirty minutes after that showed that my blood sugar levels had again returned to around the 90 points plateau.

During such fasts, one tends to become reflective. I wondered to myself just how it was that I could live on orange juice, which is mostly a mildly acidic dose of sugar water, and yet all of my diabetic symptoms would disappear. I wondered why my best efforts at moderate eating during the rest of the year left my blood sugar levels between three hundred and fifty to four hundred points, no matter if I ate garbage-foods or if

I ate healthy foods. I knew that I was on to something, but I could not figure it out for another decade. But the answer to my riddles was there before me the entire time. And during a more recent fast, the whole matter began to open before my eyes.

What I had already concluded was that I would not be diabetic while on liquid diets, and that I would have the usual symptoms return only after I resumed eating regular foods. My understanding was that the body dealt differently with solid food meals as opposed to liquid meals. It quickly dawned on me that the stomach must not be adding hydrochloric acid to the already liquefied contents of the stomach while living exclusively on orange juice.

I thereby concluded that the stomach's acid was poisoning the body in diabetics. I thought about this for a long time. Could diabetes be caused by acidosis?

Three years ago, I was repairing an appliance for a nurse, and we began to discuss diabetes. I told her my ideas and my opinions were well received. I then asked her about how the intestines could handle so much acid and she replied that the small intestines were very alkaline, and that the alkalinity neutralized the acid in the food that dropped down from the stomach into the intestines. In mere moments, it all made sense to me.

Apparently, when solid food descends into the stomach, the stomach is able to determine the amount of food, and adds hydrochloric acid in the correct amount needed to completely break down the food. After a while, the valve (called the duodenum) located between the stomach and the small intestines opens and allows the now highly acidic and pulverized, liquefied food material to drop. The presence of enough alkalinity in the upper small intestines neutralizes the acidity, allowing the liquefied nutrients to be processed and absorbed through the walls of the small intestines – right into the blood stream.

Well, that is what happens to non-diabetics. The situation is very different for type two diabetics. When the valve opens and the food drops from the stomach down into the small intestines, in diabetics, there is not enough alkalinity to neutralize all of that acidity of large meals. Hence, highly acidic liquefied food matter in diabetic people overwhelms the small amount of alkalinity in the small intestines, and still being highly acidic, the nutrients enter the bloodstream.

Here, the damage begins.

When the blood becomes acidic, the cells, in order to protect themselves, stop allowing the entry of the nutrients and sugars from the blood, for the high acidity would cause great damage. The body's cells therefore begin to starve. But just in time, the body's back-up alkalinity producer adds alkalinity directly to the bloodstream, and an hour or two after the meal was consumed, the blood's acidity is neutralized, at which time the cells begin again to accept the nutrients and the sugars from the bloodstream. Biological normalcy is restored.

It was at this point of understanding that I had to do a little homework. Up to this point, most of my discoveries were logical conclusions which followed from personal experimentation. My first question was, "what caused the small intestines to become alkaline?" An online search revealed that the alkalinity was from bicarbonate produced within the pancreas. What a shocker that was!

It turns out to my complete surprise that over 90% of the pancreas is dedicated to the production of bicarbonate (effectively baking soda!) whereas only 2% of the pancreas is dedicated to the production of insulin. Nothing could have prepared me for this fact. Bicarbonate is highly alkaline, and this is how the body deals with all that stomach acid.

Therefore, we may surmise with confidence that type two diabetes is effectively acidosis of the bloodstream caused by a failure of the pancreas to adequately provide bicarbonate (alkalinity) to the upper area of the small intestines.

Further study revealed that the body's emergency acid neutralizing system comes from the kidneys. Yes, the kidneys also produce bicarbonate, but this time, it goes directly into the bloodstream. When the pancreas fails and the bloodstream becomes highly acidic, the kidneys take up the task of neutralizing the blood.

I thought that this was the end of the matter, but there is another problem that has not been addressed here: What makes the pancreas fail to provide or deliver the needed bicarbonate? It turns out that the diabetic's pancreas does still provide a small amount of bicarbonate, but that it cannot determine how much alkalinity is needed at any given time. In a type two diabetic person, the pancreas is a paralyzed, or more accurately a zombified organ.

In a non-diabetic person, the stomach signals the pancreas regarding the amount of acidity that is coming to the intestines, so the pancreas is prepared to deliver an adequate dose of bicarbonate when it is needed. In a type two diabetic person, the otherwise fully operational pancreas is in essence unable to receive the message sent by the stomach. The pancreas remains unaware of the presence of food in the stomach and therefore, the acidity will not be matched with an appropriate amount of alkalinity.

Effectively just idling, the pancreas rather blindly adds a very small amount of bicarbonate to the small intestines, an amount totally insufficient to deal with the approaching acidic onslaught which comes with every large meal. It is thus the inability of a fully functional pancreas to perform its most vital task (adequate bicarbonate delivery) which causes the complications which diabetic people experience.

The question arises, "Why does the pancreas of a type two diabetic not perform correctly?" The answer is that the pancreas is partially paralyzed, almost certainly by food sensitivity to grains; to all grains.

It is my hope that diabetic research might partially be refocused on the effects of grains on the functionality of the pancreas. If this proves to be the culprit, efforts might be made to discover which enzyme or other factor present in food grains causes this problem. We might then either modify the grains to eliminate this factor, or we might find a means by which the pancreas loses its sensitivity to grains. By either means, diabetes can be eradicated worldwide and forever.

Doctors have often told type two diabetics that if they would lose the weight, the patient would lose the diabetes. Yet if this is new approach is correct, then it is not the weight loss that eliminates the diabetes, it is the act of dieting itself.

As we have earlier stated, the pancreas of a diabetic person cannot know how much alkalinity to put in the small intestines, but the pancreas (blindly) does add small amounts of bicarbonate to the small intestines all of the time. So when a diabetic begins to lose weight by dieting, the size of the meals is greatly reduced. The stomach recognizes that the meals are very small, so it only adds a very small amount of acid to the food.

When the slightly acidic, liquefied food drops into the small intestines, there is adequate alkalinity present, so the acidity becomes neutralized. The pH balanced blood allows the cells to accept the nutrients and sugars from the blood. Diabetes effectively disappears and remains gone until the person abandons the diet, regardless of how much weight was lost. At the conclusion of the dieting period, the meals will increase in size and the amount of acidity added to the food will increase, returning the full gamut of diabetic symptoms and complications.

Recent advances in weight loss brought about by the technique known as lap band surgery have added verification to this theory. After lap band surgery, morbidly obese people are forced to greatly restrict the amount of food in each meal. Again, a smaller stomach results in smaller meals which require very little acid, which can be adequately neutralized by the limited, but now sufficient amount of highly alkaline bicarbonate.

It is a big story in the medical world that people who undergo lap band surgery cease to be diabetics within weeks, and nobody can figure out why. How can it be that people who weigh over five hundred pounds are able to lose the diabetes before losing the morbid obesity?

This goes against everything being taught for a hundred years. When diabetes is viewed from the conventional sugar/insulin paradigm, these results make no sense. But when viewed from an acidity/alkalinity approach to diabetes, this lap band surgical consequence is completely predictable and understandable. The advice to diabetic patients, "lose the weight, lose the diabetes" could be much more accurately restated, "shrink the meals, lose the diabetes even before you lose the weight." It's not the weight, and it never really was about the weight.

Now, regarding symptoms, we can approach the matter in an entirely new light: Why do diabetics go blind? Because the eyes are being bathed in acid. Why do kidneys fail? They are being bathed in acid. Why do so many diabetics suffer from diverticulitis and diverticulosis? Because the stomach acid pours directly into that part of the small intestines with every large meal. Why do diabetics so often die from heart failure? Because the heart muscles must work ceaselessly even though the acidity of the blood so often prevents the cells of the heart muscles from gaining proper nourishment. One by one, the heart cells die of starvation or exhaustion. In time, a weakened heart can work no more and stops functioning.

Now to an even more somber topic: comas. Recall that when the meal is being processed, the bloodstream is overwhelmed with high acidity. The cells effectively close themselves off from their only source of nutrients and the blood's sugar. Cells run on sugar. When a meal is being processed, if the cells refuse to consume the sugars and nutrients present in the blood due to acidosis, it is only natural that the sugar level of the blood must remain high.

The starving cells dare not accept the dangerously acidic blood products. But at some point, the kidneys secrete bicarbonate into the blood stream, and within minutes, the cells, all of the body's cells, go from starving to gorging, taking in as much sugar and nutrients as possible, and all at once.

What does this do to blood sugar levels? The recently high (untouched) sugars in the blood stream become ingested and are consumed by all of the cells, resulting in a sudden and dangerous decrease in blood sugar levels. If the diabetic person followed the usual medical advice to avoid sugary foods and desserts, then the body's demands for sugar is unable to be fulfilled. The diabetic person's blood sugar level goes from alarmingly high to alarmingly low in minutes as the cells gorge. Lacking sugars, the diabetic person is susceptible to go into diabetic shock, coma and death. Should have had that apple pie.

Obedient diabetic patients all too often have these complications. It makes little sense when viewed from a sugar/insulin point of view, but when seen from an acidity/alkalinity perspective, the things which result in comas are both easily understandable and suddenly completely preventable.

In conclusion, it is the author's opinion, based on a lifetime of study and individual self-experimentation, that type two diabetes is not so much a matter of sugar, weight and insulin, but a disaster brought about by a pancreas that delivers too little alkalinity to the small intestines. This occurs because the pancreas is stunned and unresponsive due to a specific sensitivity to grain products.

My focus for my own self-treatment includes the need to decrease the intake of grain products and to additionally reduce the size of my meals.

Regarding the medical establishment, it is hoped that some research might be directed towards discovering why certain people have grain sensitivities, and to discover what element present in grain products trigger the pancreas's devastating reaction. With the efforts by individuals under proper medical supervision to control the meal sizes, and with medical schools working on grains and sensitivities, it might be hoped that diabetes can be better controlled and hopefully eliminated in a generation.

CHAPTER TWO

THE PANCREAS, INSULIN AND BLOOD SUGAR

The above is sufficient to know what we are dealing with and what we ought to be doing for diabetes care, prevention; as medical research moves ever closer towards creating a future free of diabetes. But allow me to continue, for great misunderstandings exist. It behooves researchers to understand what we've gotten right and historically, where we went wrong.

Let us briefly discuss the pancreas.

The pancreas is an organ which is located right behind the stomach. It is located there for a reason. The pancreas has multiple functions which are essential to a healthy life. For the purposes of this book, we will concentrate on two functions: the pro-duction of insulin and the production of bicarbonate.

Only about two percent of the pancreas is dedicated to the production of insulin, a hormone which makes it possible for the cells to absorb and process sugars taken from the bloodstream. The insulin production is performed by very small cell clusters called the "Islets of Langerhans".

For decades, it was believed that type two diabetics had high blood sugar levels due to a shortage of insulin. There have been ways to test blood sugar levels for a very long time, and since diabetics almost always tested high for sugars, it was a natural but erroneous conclusion that an increase in insulin would effectively cure diabetes. Millions of people have therefore been injected with often high levels of insulin in an attempt to lower the blood sugar level, as if a high level of sugar in the bloodstream was the damning factor of diabetes.

In a type two diabetic person, there is not an excess of sugar in the body, but there is a detectably high level of sugar in the blood stream. The body loves sugar, and in fact the cells live off of sugar and nutrients. As stated earlier, the blood sugar level in a diabetic person is only high because the blood is too acidic for the cells to be able to feed themselves properly from the bloodstream. The cells are unable to pull in sugars, so of course the sugar levels in the blood stream must be unusually high.

17

There has been a way to measure blood sugar levels for ages, but the means to measure insulin levels is a much more recent development. Now that actual insulin levels are measurable, to everybody's amazement, it has been shown that in most cases, diabetics have plenty of insulin.

In a panic, medical professionals came up with a new term to explain away this phenomenon: "insulin resistance". Reasoning that if there was sufficient insulin in a person, but the blood sugar levels remained high, then the most obvious explanation would be that the cells somehow reject all that insulin, making it difficult for the cells to absorb and process the sugar. But the guess was wrong.

Once "insulin resistance" became the new slang term, the medical research behemoth shifted directions towards creating new chemicals that might induce the cells to accept the sugar, overcoming the "resistance" any cells might have regarding insulin. Metformin is a popular medicine today, fabricated not to increase the insulin production, but to force the cells to accept the sugar coursing through the acidified bloodstream.

Today, with careful additions of artificial insulin and drugs such as metformin, patients indeed have a degree of control of their blood sugar levels. So why is this not even close to being a cure for diabetes? Why are diabetics still sickly when they have reasonable blood sugar levels? The answer is that these approaches are merely trying to alleviate symptoms, completely missing the root cause of diabetes or allowing for better approaches to treatment and care.

As important as knowing that there are better methods of treating and perhaps eliminating diabetics, we might do well to investigate exactly when and how modern medicine first erred in thinking that it was all about sugar levels and insulin. Any book or website regarding the history of diabetes can show us the error from earlier times which locked our medical world onto the wrong path.

Note: If you detect that I do not show citations in this book, it is because all of the important discoveries in this book were performed by me alone and without any scholarly references. Only in recent weeks have I begun to read the traditional discussions about diabetes. For those scholarly gentlemen and ladies who demand citations, I state firmly here that the only place I read anything related to diabetes has been at Wikipedia.org, and the readings were only very recently and for determining a few rudimentary facts for the purpose of making the message clear.

What follows is based upon reading the history of the discovery of insulin from Wikipedia. Wikipedia.org is hardly a respectable source for information in academia, but this book was not written in a university nor particularly for university researchers. If the reader wishes to do further research, I suggest a personal inquiry be undertaken completely apart from this book or from my one cited source.

Back to our topic: "When did we go so wrong?"

Now, a long citation (with my apologies) from Wikipedia.org:

In 1869, while studying the structure of the pancreas under a microscope, Paul Langerhans, a medical student in Berlin, identified some previously unnoticed tissue clumps scattered throughout the bulk of the pancreas. The function of the "little heaps of cells", later known as the *islets of Langerhans*, initially remained unknown, but Edouard Laguesse later suggested they might produce secretions that play a regulatory role in digestion. Paul Langerhans' son, Archibald, also helped to understand this regulatory role. The term "insulin" originates from *insula*, the Latin word for islet/island.

In 1889, the Polish-German physician Oscar Minkowski, in collaboration with Joseph von Mering, removed the pancreas from a healthy dog to test its assumed role in digestion. Several days after the removal of the dog's pancreas, Minkowski's animal-keeper noticed a swarm of flies feeding on the dog's urine. On testing the urine, they found sugar, establishing for the first time a relationship between the pancreas and diabetes. In 1901 Eugene Lindsay Opie took another major step forward when he clearly established the link between the islets of Langerhans and diabetes: "Diabetes mellitus . . . is caused by destruction of the islets of Langerhans and occurs only when these bodies are in part or wholly destroyed". Before Opie's work, medical science had clearly established the link between the pancreas and diabetes, but not the specific role of the islets.

Does anybody see it? Allow me to explain. Langerhans discovered the cell clusters in cadaver pancreases. Minkowski and Mering removed a pancreas and the dog became diabetic. Later Opie correctly showed the relationship between the cell clusters called the Islets of Langerhans and diabetes, but note: Opie stated firmly that:

""Diabetes mellitus . . . is caused by destruction of the islets of Langerhans and occurs only when these bodies are in part or wholly destroyed" (See citation above)

That one sentence is where everything went wrong. He intentionally destroyed the insulin producing cells in a pancreas. This is not how the body works. In a type two diabetic, the Islets of Langerhans have not been destroyed. With perfectly functioning Islets of Langerhans, hundreds of millions of people are still diabetic today.

Researcher Eugene Lindsay Opie did not realize that in diabetic people, the Islets of Langerhans were actively producing insulin, as his method (butchering the little things) was at fault. Autopsies on actual diabetics could have easily shown this to be the case. But on the authority of his word, the medical world rushed headlong into a never ending series of researches into the "insulin-deficiency causation of diabetes". To this day, type two diabetics are force-fed daily injections of insulin, and with the added insulin, diabetics receive a partial alleviation of symptoms while remaining ill for the remainder of their years.

Using blood sugar levels to determine the amount if insulin to be injected is the common practice. Since most diabetics have a normal level of insulin already, adding this powerful hormone, insulin, has its consequences. Double-dosing any hormone has consequences. Insulin injections have never cured anybody of anything, although it is a needed supplement for Type One diabetics (which is entirely outside the scope of this book).

It is commonly misunderstood that the presence of higher than average levels of sugar in the bloodstream somehow brings on all of the debilitating and irritating problems in diabetes. The actual problem is that the pancreas is failing to deliver enough bicarbonate (alkalinity) to the upper reaches of the small intestines, which causes the cells to avoid the blood's acidity, thereby blocking out the sugars and nutrients that every cell needs to sustain itself.

High blood sugar does not mean that a person has too much sugar in the body, but might indicate a lack of sugar. If the sugar remains in the blood stream, obviously there is little or none going to the cells, which is exactly where the sugar is desperately needed. Cells run on sugar.

Now a note regarding type two diabetes and heart attacks. I do not claim to know how medical professionals explain the very high rate of heart attacks among diabetics, and I do not feel the need to pore over endless articles on the topic.

From the acidosis point of view, heart attacks are completely to be expected, and here is why: The heart muscles never stop working. To survive, they must have a constant supply of nutrients, including sugar. But for diabetic people, the high acidity in the bloodstream prevents the cells from accepting nutrients. For over an hour, each cell is kept waiting for the blood acid levels to drop back to normal. Heart cells starve to death, having been forced to work ceaselessly without nourishment. At some point, the heart is so depleted of healthy muscle cells that exhaustion often results in a heart attack; an expected and tragic yet avoidable situation.

While often living entirely upon liquid diets (which I call fasting above), my stomach never detected solid foods and did not add much if any stomach acid to my liquid meals. Within days, my blood sugar dropped to very acceptable levels and all of my diabetic symptoms would disappear despite the fact that I was living on an intentionally sugary diet which often included a blender full of homemade sugary milkshakes at the end of the day.

I would consume so much liquid during such tests that I never felt hungry during the first three weeks. The few times I tried to fast beyond three weeks, my stomach let me know that enough was enough. I was really, suddenly hungry in the common under-standing of the word. Ending the fast with fresh fruit safely allowed me to resume a diet of solids.

My self-treatment could be stated thus: No solid food intake = no stomach acid being added = no blood acidosis = all evidence of diabetes vanishing.

The purpose of this small book is to provide hope for type two diabetics and hope that modern researchers will find new techniques which prevent the pancreas from failing to deliver sufficient alkalinity. This book is additionally written to inform diabetics that dietary modifications (grain-avoidance, reduction of meal size) can bring tremendous relief from the debilitating effects of diabetes.

This message is for informational purposes only, and I do not suggest any course of action without first consulting a medical professional. I don't consult doctors, but I of course suggest that everybody else should. (See disclaimer)

It is my hope that should medical investigators consider this new approach, much suffering might be alleviated, perhaps leading to new treatments and techniques to mitigate the damaging effects of diabetes.

CHAPTER THREE

DON'T TRY THIS AT HOME

Because of the weirdness of the laws in this country, it is ill advised that I suggest that anybody take actions regarding health based upon what I write here. I not only do not wish for people to act based upon the contents of this book, I strongly urge everybody to do nothing based upon this book. Just read and ponder.

I do not wish to instruct people about what to do regarding the proper manner for managing their own lives. Rather, and for legal reasons which might incur heavy penalties, I prefer to only mention the things I have done and the things that have greatly aided me in my own health quest.

As for myself, when I eat a few donuts, I feel terrible for several hours. In my youth, I blamed the sugar, whereas, today I blame the donut itself. It is made from a grain product. In the past, I would normally only eat a donut when I was hungry, so in essence, I was consuming processed grain on an empty stomach. The pancreas would be stunned, the blood sugar would be remaining high, and I would struggle to function normally, feeling weighted down far beyond what one would expect from such a light meal.

This week, as a delicious experiment, I consumed five pancakes, adding plenty of artificially sweetened syrup. For the entire day, I was light headed, short tempered and felt miserable. If we cannot blame the sugar-free syrup, how do we explain this? It's the grain product, the pancakes themselves, that so ruined my day.

As a type two diabetic, I can receive partial alleviation of symptoms when I consume meat products along with grain products. It might be simply that the meat slows the digestion, allowing the grain products to process more slowly. The sudden jolt of a donut on an empty stomach can be disconcerting, while spaghetti with meatballs usually is not. A cheeseburger processes better than buttered toast.

Over the decades, my personal self-experimentation has taught me these things:

On days in which I avoid grain products, I usually feel better than when I consume them. During weeks in which I minimize grain products, I usually feel energetic, and many of my diabetic symptoms will significantly decrease in severity. During weeks in which I live entirely on liquids, my blood sugar drops to normal levels, I feel energetic, and most or all diabetic complications disappear until I return to a regular American foods diet.

The key factors in my experience are meal size (which adds stomach acid) and/or the amount of grain products consumed (increasing paralysis of the pancreas).

I no longer try to avoid sugar, although I do try to eat healthier foods. In my regular existence, I usually consume one or two pounds of fresh grapes each day, as I find them delicious. I do not worry about how much sugar it might add to my diet. Sugar, for me, is not all that important a factor. In my experience, if processed sugar is especially harmful, it is probably only after the pancreas is damaged by grain products.

That some sugar is derived from sugar cane is a concern. Sugar cane, like wheat, rice and oats, is from a family of grasses. I do not know if this is a factor, but that is for others to figure out. For myself, fruit sugars and honey are my personal favorites, and I do not avoid them in the least.

Questions? Comments? Complaints? Feel free to contact the author via email:

rethinkdiabetes@aol.com

www.ingramcontent.com/pod-product-compliance
Lightning Source LLC
Chambersburg PA
CBHW031221290326
41931CB00035B/663